# 12 TOP BEST CANCER FIGHTING FOOD

## Unveiling the right kind of food to stop cancer spreads

By

Dr DOUGLAS JASON

Copyright © (DR DOUGLAS JASON) 2023. All rights reserved

Before this document is duplicated or reproduced in any manner, the publisher's consent must be gained.

Therefore, the contents within can neither be stored electronically, transferred, nor kept in a database. Neither in part nor in full can the document be copied, scanned, faxed, or retained without approval from the publisher or creator.

**TABLE OF CONTENT**

**ABOUT THE AUTHOR**

**INTRODUCTION**

**TABLE OF CONTENTS**

## 12 TOP BEST CANCER FIGHTING FOOD

## Unveiling the right kind of food to stop cancer

## INTRODUCTION

## CHAPTER 1
## USING COLOR TO FIGHT CANCER

## CHAPTER 2
## CANCER-FIGHTING BREAKFAST (FOLATE)

## CHAPTER 3
## Pass Up the Deli Counter.

CHAPTER 4
CANCER-FIGHTING TOMATOES.

CHAPTER 5
The Anticancer Potential of GREEN Tea

CHAPTER 6
Grapes and Cancer

CHAPTER 7
CLEAN WATER

CHAPTER 8
The Mighty Bean

CHAPTER 9
The Cabbage Family.

**CHAPTER 10**
**Dark-green Leafy Vegetables**

**CHAPTER 11**
**Defense Against an Exotic Spice.**

**CHAPTER 12**
**BERRIES FAMILY WITH A PUNCH,**

**CONCLUSION**

## ABOUT THE AUTHOR

Dr. Douglas Jason is a certified dietician who has a strong passion for wellness and a big eagerness to help people all over the world. He uses healthy food, herbs, spices, and other useful tools to help mankind realize its overall goal of optimum health.

# INTRODUCTION

Fighting Cancer by the Plateful Cancer cannot be prevented by a single diet, but the appropriate food combinations may assist. At mealtimes, aim for a balance of no more than one-third animal protein and at least two-thirds plant-based foods. According to the American Institute for Cancer Research, this "New American Plate" is a crucial aid in the fight against cancer. Examine the best and worst options for your plate.

# CHAPTER 1

# USING COLOR TO FIGHT CANCER

Cancer-preventing nutrients are abundant in fruits and vegetables, and the more color a food has, the more nutrition it has. When you achieve and keep a healthy body weight, these meals can also reduce your risk in another way. Obesity raises the risk of several malignancies, such as colon, esophageal, and kidney cancers. Consume a diversity of veggies, focusing on those that are dark green, red, and orange.

# CHAPTER 2

# CANCER-FIGHTING BREAKFAST (FOLATE)

Natural folate is a crucial B vitamin that may help prevent malignancies of the breast, colon, and rectum. On the breakfast table, there is a ton of stuff. Good sources of folate include whole wheat products and breakfast cereals that have been fortified. Likewise, strawberries, melons, and orange juice.

Asparagus and eggs are two additional excellent sources of folate. Additionally, it is present in legumes, sunflower seeds, and leafy greens like romaine lettuce and spinach. Not from a pill, but eating enough fruits, vegetables, and items made with enriched grains, is the greatest method to obtain folate. To ensure that they obtain enough folic acid to help prevent some birth defects, women who are pregnant or may become pregnant should take a supplement.

# CHAPTER 3

## Pass Up the Deli Counter.

You won't get sick from the occasional Reuben sandwich or hot dog at the stadium. However, reducing your consumption of processed meats like hot dogs, ham, and bologna will help reduce your risk of colorectal and stomach cancer. Additionally, eating meats that have been salted or smoked increases your exposure to chemicals that may one day lead to cancer.

# CHAPTER 4

# CANCER-FIGHTING TOMATOES.

It's unclear whether the cause is lycopene, the ingredient that gives tomatoes their red color, or something else. However, some research suggests that consuming tomatoes may lessen your risk of developing certain cancers, including prostate cancer. Additionally, studies indicate that processed tomato products like juice, sauce or paste have a higher capacity to fight cancer.

# CHAPTER 5

# The Anticancer Potential of GREEN Tea

Tea, especially green tea, maybe a potent cancer fighter, albeit the evidence is currently fragmentary. Green tea has been shown to reduce or stop the growth of prostate, colon, liver, and breast cancer in laboratory experiments. Similar results were seen in skin and lung tissue as well. Additionally, in certain longer-term trials, tea consumption was linked to a reduced incidence of pancreatic, stomach, and bladder cancer. However, further human studies are required before tea can be suggested as a cancer preventative.

# CHAPTER 6

# Grapes and Cancer

Resveratrol is found in grapes and grape juice, particularly in purple and red grapes. Strong anti-inflammatory and antioxidant effects are seen in resveratrol. In laboratory tests, it has stopped the type of cell damage that can start the cancerous process. The possibility that eating grapes, drinking grape juice or wine, or taking supplements can either prevent or treat cancer is not supported by sufficient data.

To reduce the risk of cancer, limit alcohol consumption.

Alcohol consumption has been associated with cancers of the mouth, throat, larynx, esophagus, liver, and breast. The risk of colon and rectum cancer may also increase with alcohol consumption. Although the American Cancer Society advises against drinking, if you do, try to keep your intake to no more than two drinks per day for males and one drink per day for women. According to their risk factors, women who are more likely to develop breast cancer may want to consult a doctor about how much alcohol, if any, is safe to consume.

# CHAPTER 7
# CLEAN WATER

Fluids Can Protect, such as Water. In addition to quenching your thirst, water may also help prevent bladder cancer. Water dilutes the concentrations of probable cancer-causing chemicals in the bladder, lowering the risk. Additionally, you urinate more frequently when you drink more fluids. As a result, those substances come into contact with the bladder lining for a shorter period.

# CHAPTER 8

# The Mighty Bean

Given how healthy beans are, it should come as no surprise that they may also aid in the fight against cancer. They include several powerful phytochemicals that might shield the body's cells from harm that could cause cancer. In the lab, these compounds inhibited tumor release of chemicals that harm neighboring cells and halted tumor growth.

# CHAPTER 9

## The Cabbage Family.

Broccoli, cauliflower, cabbage, Brussels sprouts, bok choy, and kale are examples of cruciferous vegetables. These cabbage family members make fantastic stir-fries and can truly enliven a salad. Most importantly, however, is that certain elements in these vegetables may support your body's defense mechanisms against malignancies like colon, breast, lung, and cervix. Although human trials have yielded mixed outcomes, laboratory research has proved promising.

# CHAPTER 10

## Dark-green Leafy Vegetables

Dark green leafy vegetables are rich in fiber, folate, and carotenoids. Examples include mustard greens, lettuce, kale, chicory, spinach, and chard. These vitamins and minerals may offer defense against stomach, skin, lung, larynx, mouth, and pancreatic cancer.

# CHAPTER 11

## Defense Against an Exotic Spice.

The primary component of the Indian spice turmeric, curcumin, may be able to combat cancer. It can prevent a variety of malignancies from transforming, proliferating, and invading, according to laboratory research. Human research is still being done.

# CHAPTER 12

# BERRIES FAMILY WITH A PUNCH,

Ellagic acid is a phytochemical found in strawberries and raspberries. This potent antioxidant may combat cancer by delaying the growth of cancer cells and destroying several chemicals that cause the disease. However, there isn't enough evidence to claim that it can treat cancer in people just yet.

The strong antioxidants found in blueberries may be beneficial for many aspects of human health, beginning with cancer. By removing free radicals from the body before they can harm cells, antioxidants may help fight cancer. However, more study is required. To increase your intake of these beneficial berries, try adding blueberries to oatmeal, cold cereal, yogurt, and even salad.

## CONCLUSION

The amount of cancer risk that meat carries can vary depending on how it is prepared. Meats that have been fried, grilled, or broiled at extremely high temperatures form compounds that may raise the risk of cancer. Stewing, braising, or steaming appear to produce less of those toxins than other cooking techniques. And when you simmer the meat, don't forget to include a lot of wholesome vegetables.

omit the sugar.
Cancer may not be directly caused by sugar. However, it might replace

other nutrient-rich foods that aid in cancer prevention. Additionally, it raises calorie intake, which plays a part in obesity and being overweight. Cancer risks can include being overweight. Fruit provides a healthy sweet alternative that is also vitamin-rich.

Avoid depending on supplements Vitamins may aid in cancer prevention. However, that is when you naturally obtain them from meals. The American Cancer Society and the American Institute for Cancer Research both highlight that eating foods like nuts, fruits, and green leafy vegetables instead of taking supplements is by far the best way to obtain nutrients that prevent cancer. The best diet is a nutritious one.

www.ingramcontent.com/pod-product-compliance
Lightning Source LLC
Chambersburg PA
CBHW050324220526
45465CB00005B/2116